"Yeeks!"

GETTING SAFELY THROUGH PERIMENOPAUSE, MENOPAUSE AND BEYOND

HELEN GRECO, MD
JANE RABIN STERN

This book could not have been written without the understanding and sense of humor of our families. Thank you Joseph, Stephanie, and Thomas, and Russell, Florence and Robert. We love you very much.

Acknowledgements

We express our appreciation to Dr. Vicki L. Seltzer, Vice President for Women's Health Services, North Shore Long Island Jewish Health System, Chairman, Departments of Obstetrics and Gynecology, Long Island Jewish Medical Center and North Shore University Hospital, whose dedication to women's health has been an inspiration.

Thanks to Nancy Cohen Farber, Nurse Practitioner, for providing research assistance, Cathy Aronna Campbell for her technical help, Gerald Boshi for his encouragement from the start, and The Partners in Women's Health for their ongoing support.

Procedes from the sale of this book will benefit the Ann and Jules Gottlieb Women's Comprehensive Health Center of the North Shore Long Island Jewish Health System.

This book is dedicated to
Judy R. Goldsmith

Contents

Introduction

Introduction

What I want to do is empower women to control their own health and destiny.

This is for all women who really want to take care of themselves. I want to educate them, and learning through this book is a fun way for them to do that.

I want women to understand their bodies, to know, what does a breast look like? What do my ovaries look like? Where is estrogen coming from? What is my hypothalamus? Why do I feel the hot flashes in my face and you tell me it's all in my brain? What has estrogen to do with that? How does everything work?

Really, if women read this book, it will benefit them to have this information.

The patients I see are so pleased to be offered different ideas and options, whether it is to go on hormones or not to go on hormones, or just to understand what their bodies are going through. I would like all women to know these things.

A lot of women have troubles. Women can have a lot of problems in their lives because everybody else comes first and they come last. Whether it's their parents getting older, their teenagers getting into trouble, their husbands, whatever it is, they get sidetracked. They let things go in terms of taking care of themselves.

I just want to give them some information to learn in a nice way, with facts, stories and different images.

I want them to be able to read about what makes them

comfortable, besides being healthy!

I think most women should feel rested and happy, and content for what they can control.

There are a lot of things in our lives that we cannot control. We cannot change people, but we can change ourselves and our own outlook on how to handle different stresses. You see how stress affects your body, it can put people way down.

When I take care of my patients, I want them to feel good about themselves. Walk around with a smile!

Patients of mine have said, "You have a way of thinking, you come up with good ideas." And it's true that I like to guide them into being able to handle their own situations. After seeing me they should walk out feeling "I can do this. I can take care of myself." And it's not just trusting a physician, it's being responsible for your own care.

Maybe at this time in a woman's life she has to find new roles and ways to make herself happy, maybe new interests or hobbies.

It's not just a question of taking pills!

I want a woman to learn about her options, and feel that she is in control.

When a woman has a happy or contented outlook she feels better about herself. This is not just a healthy attitude, it's good for you, too.

I want every woman to feel as good as she can.

1. Estrogen Bath.

Do you know we all started out as girls?

When we start out in the womb, we're all the same. We're all girls.

The sexes don't become visibly different until the 10th week of gestation. Genetically speaking, we are boys or girls. But in the womb it's all about hormones, and genetics has to wait until the hormones make a physical impression on the fetus.

During pregnancy, estrogen is produced almost exclusively from the placenta. The amount made each day during the last few weeks of pregnancy is 1000 times as much estrogen as the ovaries were making before pregnancy. Can you imagine?

This estrogen rich environment is called an estrogen bath and is ideal for female development. By the second month of gestation, the tiny ovaries of the female fetus are estimated to have already made 600,000 eggs!

But to become males, male fetuses must work like crazy to make enough testosterone from their testes to differentiate themselves. They do this, I think, because they don't want to become women!

How amazing are these hormones that can make us into boys and girls?

What this mostly affects is the hypothalamus, which is located at the base of the brain. It's a walnut-sized structure and this is what dictates the hormones for sexual development and sexual behavior. It also regulates water balance and temperature.

I don't think women realize how important estrogen is throughout our lives, starting in utero. It plays a vital role in our evolution and development!

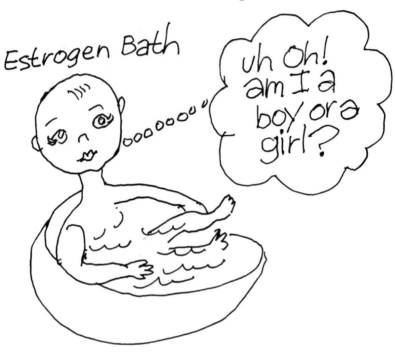

While the female fetus is still in the estrogen bath, her ovaries will have made as many as 7 million eggs! By the time she is born, these eggs, (actually they're the precursors to the eggs which will develop), are reduced in number to 2 million.

You see, our potential for reproducing slows down before we're even born, so you might think we're already going into some sort of perimenopause while we're in the womb!

Once the female baby is born, there is no more estrogen until puberty. There are only estrogen receptors. The body is smart, and shuts down estrogen production until it's fully developed, so you can't have the capability to reproduce until your body is grown.

By the time of puberty there are about 1/2 million eggs left, and during the reproductive years, just 400-500 will actually be ovulated.

Then after a time a woman's capability for reproducing the species ends, she stops making estrogen again. And as far as nature is concerned, although men keep making testosterone until the day they die, women weren't meant to live that long.

2. Menopause - What is it really?

It's a gradual process, but it sounds so final.

It's all about hormones, but what is going on? !

Well actually, as simply as you can put it, menopause is the last menstrual period a woman may experience. And it's something all women go through.

It seems many women get confused thinking about menopause.

Menopause is not one but a series of changes. It is all related to the decreased production of estrogen by the ovaries. Our menstrual cycles thereby become less frequent and lighter.

It marks the end of our reproductive years. Ovulation (*ova* is the Greek word for egg) occurs less often. And then, some time around an average age in the United States of 51, this process ends. But usually it does not end abruptly.

It is usually preceded by a series of changes that can last anywhere from months to years. The fluctuation in hormones can start as early as 5 years before the last period and continue for a number of years afterwards.

That's why everyone experiences menopause differently!

For some women it may be a smooth transition, and for others it may create both physical and psychological stress.

Do you remember those teenage years, with everything going up and down in your life at once? (If you don't remember, just look at any teenager today - maybe you have one of your own!)

Now think of yourself as a teenager, but only backwards!

The hormones that created havoc when they first entered our bodies are now doing the same thing as they're leaving!

If the reduction of hormones is smooth and easy, it might not be noticed very much. But if the fluctuations are wild, the symptoms may be hard to deal with. We've all seen it in others or even in ourselves. Maybe that's why menopause isn't something women look forward to.

Thin women experience menopause differently from heavy women. Heavier women make "their own" estrogen in fatty tissue, and that is why they are usually less symptomatic from menopausal symptoms such as hot flashes. They also have protection against osteoporosis. On the other hand, they are at risk for endometrial cancer because of unopposed estrogen, which I will mention later.

25% of the women in America will enter menopause suddenly for reasons relating to illness, such as surgical removal of the ovaries, chemotherapy or radiation, or from premature ovarian failure.

I think our attitude has to change so we don't just think about getting into menopause, but rather going through it safely!

When we first went through puberty, we were all very excited, at least most of us, about menstruating, getting breasts, and becoming women. Now it is a time in a woman's life for her to be enjoying herself again. We should look forward to these years and have a better attitude towards them, instead of being so afraid and confused.

At last our children tend to be more on their own, it's well past the time most women would have more children, and there's no reason to worry about contraceptives. I wonder, what could be better?

If we understood our bodies, I think we could handle this time well, and again look forward to change. If women learn how to manage menopause, it will not manage them.

Today we are expected to spend as much as a third of our lives beyond menopause, so it's extremely important to learn how to live with this new state. The best way to learn how to experience menopause is to understand it so that you can better cope with it. Estrogen or hormone replacement therapy can help with this transition, but so can exercise and diet. Good nutrition, vitamins and calcium supplements are all very important.

3. "Why do I feel this way?"

So now you know that a woman may experience changes physically and emotionally for months or even years before menopause actually occurs.

Some people refer to this time around menopause as perimenopause, and that's what the word literally means. But I don't think it explains things very well. It really is a continuum. It's a transition beginning from the time when a woman is still in her reproductive years.

We all have our plans, how we're going to go through menopause, and then something different happens!

You know why women get confused thinking about menopause? Because - doctors themselves confuse them!

Some will say, "Oh, you have to wait a whole year after your last period until you're truly in menopause." But that's not so. Changes are occurring throughout perimenopause.

Women may complain about their symptoms and they speak up more. They're not happy with answers like "Oh, don't worry about it, that's normal."

Some will even leave their doctors because their questions are not answered to their satisfaction.

Many women like to see a physician when they feel they can just say what's on their mind, and get answers like they're talking to a friend. I can give them real answers to questions like, "Why do I feel this way?" or "Why are my periods coming every three weeks?" An explanation shared with patients about why they're feeling different may help them understand better, and it becomes quite alright.

Women notice a commonality in their complaints such as anxiety and panic, or feeling unsettled. There's also a tendency for a certain type of behavior where some women overreact and have sudden outbursts. There may be interactional problems, not only at home but at work. Some may feel like they're out of control of their bodies, and their emotions. They'll find this very depressing and overwhelming. It only aggravates the situation further, especially if they've been fairly emotionally stable.

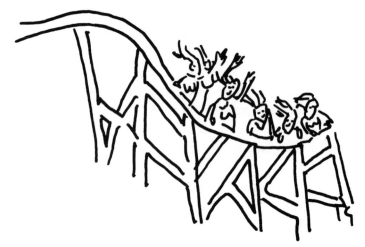

This again is very similar to what happens during adolescence. A lot depends on support at home, or in other environments. If you're feeling good about yourself, you may be able to handle these emotional changes far better than another woman who really has low self esteem, and emotionally is on a roller coaster.

But for women with a history of clinical depression, their symptoms may become aggravated or actually magnified.

This life change, because of hormonal fluctuations, is similar to other times in a woman's life cycle, such as postpartum depression, premenstrual syndrome, and puberty. Emotions can be erratic, with highs and lows and widely swinging behaviors, sometimes with periods of deep, deep sadness without a real identifiable cause. These can affect a woman's attitude about herself.

It can create a great deal of stress not only to the person herself, but also to her family and significant others.

Patients of mine tell me what's happening in their lives, and we see if we can piece together what's going on.

I go back to how women are taking care of themselves: exercise, nutrition.

I listen, and my patients know if they have something of great concern, they can discuss it with me. It's not something they have to live with by themselves and suffer quietly, if they recognize it's part of a time when priorities and levels of energy are changing.

The situation can be very difficult because of the rise and fall of levels of estrogen, sometimes a few times a day. When it's just too much, then a patient may discuss hormone replacement therapy, if medically appropriate, or other alternatives with her physician.

4. When to use hormone replacement therapy during perimenopause.

Many women in perimenopause are having a difficult time because of the fluctuating levels of estrogen that occur at this time. This can cause lack of sleep from hot flashes, then stress and other related symptoms because of that. Emotionally, what they're going through can be awful!

I have patients who are suffering so terribly emotionally that they have a hard time with their daily living. Previously they managed home or work situations fairly well and in an organized fashion. However, the strain of these changes kind of just tips some women over, it's just too much. There can be lack of concentration, fatigue, and irritability to the point of being unreasonable.

Once they get back to "normal," they're fine again!

This is where hormone replacement therapy, HRT, can be important.

Estrogen alone was the first hormone replacement therapy. It was prescribed way back in 1942. Women then wanted relief just as they do today from hot flashes, which is still the most common complaint.

I had a patient come in and her blood pressure was elevated.

"Oh, I'm so nervous when I come to see you," she said.

"Why? Little old me? I've known you for years," I replied.

"No, I'm afraid you might take my hormones away."

I said, "Why, what did you do?"

"Nothing. I'm just afraid you'd take them away. I couldn't live without them!"

Not everybody has to take hormones, but some women feel better because of them. That's the important thing. I mean it's nice to look better because you feel better. But I think women, with some of the emotional fluctuations, the moods, and then all the pressure they're having, I think this is something they should have.

Many women are mothers or professionals, or both, and with everything they do, they feel things should be black or white, with no in between. It's time to cook dinner, it's time to go to work, it's time to wash the clothes, it's time...and there's no gray, there's no flexibility, you know. And I think women who are flexible are more likely to deal with this transition a little more easily. But there are women who are inflexible and say, "I didn't plan on it!" They just can't tolerate unpredictable happenings in their body or anywhere else in their lives.

How often is the answer HRT?

I think everyone has some difficulty, but some women handle it better than others, or just have an easier time. It's important to speak to your physician.

11

Then with some women, it's quite obvious. I can hear it, they're frantic. They'll say, "My husband's so great, he's so good, and I toss and turn all night and keep him awake because of all those hot flashes..." That's the woman I usually have to give HRT to, even if she's not quite menopausal, meaning she still gets periods occasionally. And don't forget! Perimenopausal women still need contraception. They are still ovulating, although infrequently.

5. Hormones and Perimenopause.

I would say most women during perimenopause notice changes in their menstrual cycles.

It's hard to describe what goes on during a menstrual cycle in terms of hormones. They do a lot of different things, and it's very confusing.

I'd like to take a few minutes and explain this.

Changes in menstrual cycles relate to the changes in levels of estrogen. These changes affect a small walnut-sized gland in the brain called the hypothalamus. It regulates the production of hormones by the ovaries, controls our thermal regulation, and to some extent our moods. That's why everyone keeps saying that the control for the body is there, in this little walnut.

When estrogen levels decrease, the hypothalamus sends out signals that are hormonal to get the ovaries to make more estrogen. That's what a hormone does, it sends a message to another organ. Here it uses the pituitary gland as a go between, so once it receives low levels of estrogen, the hypothalamus tells the pituitary to release a stimulating hormone that will make the ovaries generate more estrogen. The work of this hormone is to stimulate the follicles in the ovaries to make more estrogen. It's called FSH, for follicle-stimulating hormone.

When the ovaries start to slow down they produce less estrogen. More and more FSH is being sent out as the need for estrogen gets greater.It just keeps stimulating, stimulating, stimulating.

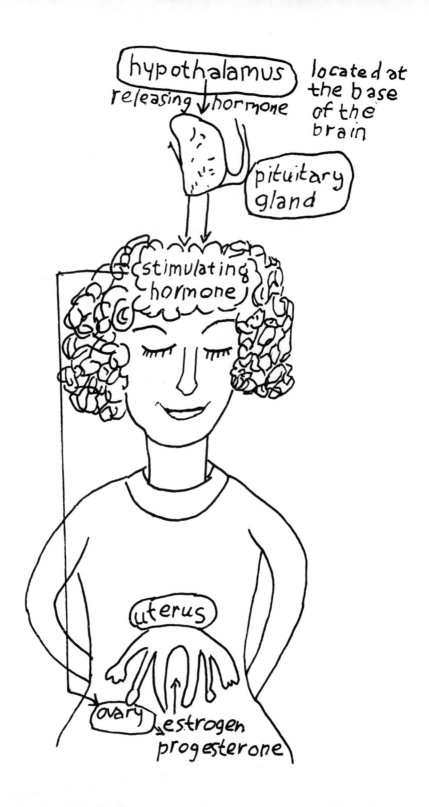

We can test levels of estrogen by measuring the levels of FSH, because the high levels of FSH are in direct response to the low levels of estrogen. Even though there's more and more FSH being sent, the ovaries simply can't make any more estrogen.

While the hypothalamus is triggering these hormonal signals, its over activity relates to the hot flashes women feel, because it's trying to regulate body temperature at the same time.

The hypothalamus also makes serotonin, epinephrine, norepinephrine, and dopamine, all substances which control moods and emotion.

So you can see what a confusing time it is for the pituitary, the hypothalamus, the ovaries, and you!

6. Hot flashes, night sweats and PMS here I come!

We've all become accustomed to hearing words like "hot flashes" and "night sweats." You hear a lot of women talking about flushes, and sweating and sleeplessness, early morning awakenings. It sounds so exhausting, and if it happens to you, you think, "There's got to be a better way!"

As a woman enters menopause there can be a number of uncomfortable physical symptoms that result from the loss of estrogen occurring at this time. Most women have some symptoms, only a few have none. As with everything else during menopause, the symptoms and their severity vary from woman to woman.

A hot flash is probably one of the most frequently reported symptoms of menopause.

It is caused by sharp drops in estrogen levels.

Hot flashes shouldn't last forever!!

The body adjusts to lack of estrogen over time. But while it does, the hypothalamus, which is reacting to this, is also controlling your thermal regulation. So that begins changing too, and that is what causes the hot flashes. A hot flash basically is the feeling of heat that begins in the chest and spreads to the neck and head, like a sudden wave across your body. It can last from a few seconds to a few minutes.

The average hot flash is usually accompanied by profuse perspiration and conspicuous reddening of the face. It can make a woman feel confused, embarrassed, helpless, bewildered and certainly self-conscious.

Some women experience hot flashes several times a day, others less frequently, and some never at all.

The uncomfortable symptoms of menopause, such as hot flashes, may continue from several months to several years. A lot of these changes can be experienced along with palpitations, wooziness, dizziness, anxiety, and even shortness of breath, panic attacks, or headaches.

In addition, these physical symptoms can produce a variety of psychological effects, many of which are related to sleep deprivation caused by night sweats.

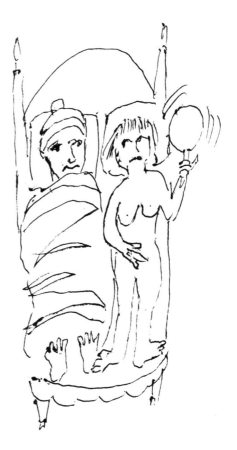

Hot flashes that occur during sleep are what we call night sweats. They may cause a woman to awaken several times during the night, with blankets and covers flung away.

Because of these disruptive night sweats, there is a

lack of sleep causing tiredness during the day.This can maximize daily stresses.

Also, a lot of perimenopausal women have aggravating PMS symptoms, some who never had PMS!

That means many women feel bloated, have tender or swollen breasts, cramps, and mood swings. They may not have had these PMS-like symptoms before, or they never really acknowledged them.

So you see how uncomfortable this time can be!

7. Perimenopause and irregular bleeding.

Entering menopause is a complicated process, and your last menstrual cycles reflect this. Bleeding can be irregular and heavy, and your periods may be different from before. You must mention this to your physician.

This is a time when it's normal to behave erratically.

For many women their biggest problem may be uncontrollable bleeding patterns. The goal really is to prevent this from happening.

It's important to go over the topic of perimenopausal periods since this irregular bleeding may also represent a serious problem.

Throughout the time before menopause, a woman's periods should be spacing themselves differently and getting lighter and lighter. However, the menstrual cycle may also become shorter since you're producing less of the hormones estrogen and progesterone. Some months you don't ovulate, and then you may miss a menstrual cycle that month.

A woman should be aware of the imbalance of hormones that occurs at this time because this can be a serious matter.

Now there may be times when you're not ovulating regularly in this time period, and again you're producing estrogen without progesterone. If there's no ovulation, then no progesterone is being produced to balance estrogen. This is called unopposed estrogen. Estrogen causes the lining of the uterus to thicken, and progesterone causes it to slough off. This is how you get a period!

To avoid a potential problem caused by the imbalance of estrogen and progesterone, a woman requires annual or even more frequent gynecologic evaluation.

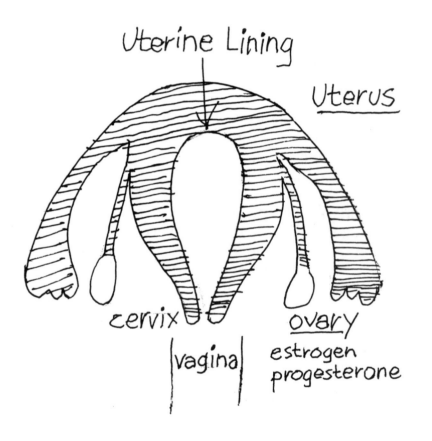

Since estrogen is a growth hormone, it can thereby stimulate the growth of uterine fibroids, especially if production of progesterone is minimal. Fibroids can cause irregular bleeding and pain.

Uterine fibroids can be in three places: on the surface of the uterus (serosal), in the muscle of the uterus (intramural), and in the lining of the uterus (submucosal). Those in the lining tend to bleed.

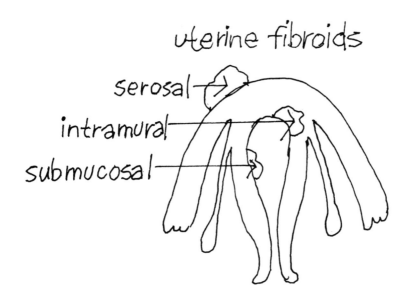

uterine fibroids

serosal

intramural

submucosal

In addition, there can be polyps in the uterine lining. That's another type of growth, and they, too, can bleed.

When there is unusual or irregular bleeding during menopause, you can't assume it's normal. You must mention it to your physician.

8. Sometimes you have to interfere to help nature run its course.

It is important to know that hormones are changing during perimenopause, and to realize that unopposed estrogen puts a woman at risk for endometrial cancer. If there's just estrogen and no progesterone, we have to watch out for that.

In a way, all of what happens naturally during this time may put us at risk. That's the normal evolution of menopause. That's why a woman at this time in her life should be under the care of a physician.

In order to evaluate abnormal bleeding patterns, an endometrial biopsy may be performed. This is when tissue is taken from the lining of the uterus, enabling us to see if the problem could be uterine cancer, or pre-cancerous changes known as hyperplasia.

An endometrial biopsy also reflects the hormonal status of the uterine lining.

A pelvic sonogram may be recommended. This is a type of radiological image of the uterus and ovaries.

Perimenopausal bleeding can be quite profuse at this time, as well as prolonged. A woman may feel weak, tired, in fact quite run down. She may be anemic.

After a thorough gynecologic evaluation, there are a number of options in managing this particular problem without necessarily performing a hysterectomy. Although don't get me wrong. In certain circumstances, a hysterectomy may be an option.

There are a number of ways hormonally to manipulate a woman's body, correct this abnormal bleeding, and ease the transition through menopause. The use of birth control pills is one example of this. As always, diet, vitamins and exercise are important, too.

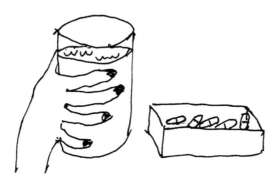

There are a lot of remarkable things in medicine today, and we can use them to give nature a helping hand.

9. "Am I ever going to stop having my period?"

A 51-year-old patient came to see me after her previous doctor put her on hormone replacement therapy to treat irregular periods and hot flashes.

She asked me, "Am I ever going to stop having my period?"

I said, "Well, I don't even know if you're menopausal yet, since your doctor put you on a cyclical regimen of hormone replacement therapy. You may be having withdrawal bleeding because of that, or you really still might be getting your own menstrual cycles here and there. So I can't even tell you if you need contraception."

"Oh, I didn't think of that!"

The doctor she was seeing just said, "You're having hot flashes and irregular periods, so go on hormones!"

I then told her, "Well, I think it's a good idea to know if you're menopausal or not, so you can decide about contraception and evaluate other health related concerns."

The thing is, she doesn't want to keep getting her period if she really is menopausal.

She didn't even realize that this particular regimen of hormone replacement gave her a period. She was never offered a choice, or told of different regimens of hormone replacement that she could take that might not bring on a period!

Taking estrogen for four weeks, and progesterone for two out of those four weeks would mimic a menstrual cycle with a withdrawal bleed. Another regimen could be a combination of estrogen and progesterone every single day, in a continuous dosage, to prevent withdrawal bleeding.

I suggested she stop the hormone replacement therapy in order to assess her baseline ovarian function better.

A woman should discuss these choices with her physician, learn about them, and make an educated decision.

10. Hormone replacement therapy. How did it all begin?

When estrogen replacement therapy was first introduced, it was to treat symptoms of menopause. These included hot flashes and vaginal dryness.

Well guess what?

Do you know that today estrogen is one of the most widely prescribed drugs for women in America?

Estrogen is given now in conjunction with progesterone, because if you have a uterus you cannot take just estrogen alone, otherwise your risk of uterine cancer is increased.

The combinatin of estrogen and progesterone is called hormone replacement therapy (HRT).

There are women who are very happy to be taking HRT. There are pros and cons talked about, but because of the media confusion, there is uncertainty about what to do. It is essential that you discuss your concerns with a physician who knows your risk factors versus the benefits.

A funny thing, when estrogen alone was first introduced, it presented itself as a sort of miracle drug, something that would keep women young forever.

Postmenopausal women had been depicted as old women. They were pictured as asexual and unattractive. Well, you don't necessarily get that way.

We all started out wrinkled and unattractive the day we were born!

Women still want to look young, but are also concerned about their health, and prevention of disease.

Now when you're in menopause, the ovaries have stopped producing estrogen. The hypothalamus is trying to stimulate the pituitary which is trying to stimulate the ovaries and they say, "I give up, this is it for me. It's gone, so it doesn't matter what you do, it's not going to work out!"

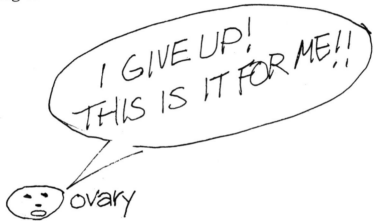

Once ovarian function is gone, the ovaries cannot produce estrogen anymore, no matter how strong the signals are from the hypothalamus and pituitary gland.

This is why the dose of estrogen in HRT is so much lower than that in birth control pills. The estrogen in hormone replacement therapy is the lowest dose that can be given safely to prevent heart disease and osteoporosis. The higher dose of estrogen in birth control pills suppresses the signals from the hypothalamus and the pituitary so that the ovaries do not ovulate, thereby providing contraception! This is no longer the goal in menopause.

It's also true that before menopause, women have a much lower rate of heart disease than men, but once estrogen is lost, their risk becomes greater. Recent studies have been done to determine to what extent long-term estrogen use may protect against heart disease, by far the leading cause of death in women.

I mentioned that hormones are not for everyone, and every woman has to make an individual decision with the assistance of a physician who has examined her.

The reason this is important is that if a woman is unhappy taking a medication, it will only distress her further to continue taking it.

She may find that switching to a regimen of exercise, good diet, calcium supplementation and a multivitamin may help her feel better about herself. She may not really want to be putting anything quote unquote foreign in her body. She does not realize that estrogen replacement is just providing what she naturally is supposed to have but at a lower dose, just enough to prevent the untoward effects of the lack of estrogen.

I think all women should learn about this for themselves, and then, with their physicians, make their own choices.

11. Hormone replacement therapy. It's not for everyone, you know.

So menopause is experienced differently in each woman and affects various systems in the body in a variety of ways.

Hormone replacement therapy is not necessary for everyone.

It must be individualized in that risks weighed against benefits must be thoroughly examined in consultation with a physician.

Each and every woman has a choice.

For example, some women on hormone replacement therapy say they experience weight gain. I have to tell them at this time in their life, it's probably happening anyway. The body is changing, and so is your metabolism, as well as the fat proportion and distribution in your body.

Menopause brings special health considerations. You may want to make some lifestyle modifications to adjust to these changes.

What's very important for a woman to understand is that all the benefits of taking HRT disappear as soon as she stops taking it!

If the concern is osteoporosis, a woman has to know that bones will begin to lose bone mass density as soon as the estrogen levels drop. The same is true for protection against heart disease. You need to be taking estrogen to get the benefits from it.

Women should ask questions, especially now, at this time in their lives. They should expect to get reasonable answers. They shouldn't just be told, "You're going through changes and that's why you need to be on HRT!"

There are all sorts of pressures placed on women at this time. There's confusion. It's all a bit scary and overwhelming.

It's not fair because women may have friends who are on HRT, and I hear, "A lot of my friends are on this and I'm not!"

Or, "My husband doesn't think I have much of a libido, but I feel fine!"

Quite often women feel comfortable going through menopause and they've been feeling okay. Then they feel pressure all around them, especially with what's in the media.

Because I have women who'll say, "You know everybody's on HRT. I read about it. Do I need to be on it? What's your advice?"

I will say, "Well, it's not my decision. This is the information, you need to think about it first. You have to decide what's best for you. "

You know a pill is not going to change your lifestyle.

You have to change that on your own anyway. It's

behavior modification with a good diet and exercise. If you feel like you're doing well, you don't have to be on HRT. Not everybody needs to be on it.

We have to maintain ourselves. We have to stay healthy, safe, and in control!

12. Why are *you* taking it?

I have a patient who has been on HRT, and every time she has a mammogram it is an ordeal. It's a problem because her breasts are so dense. This can happen on HRT.

So she sees a colleague of mine who says, "This is the second time this has happened. Why don't you get off HRT and go on a medication that won't change your breast tissue but will take care of osteoporosis? Oh, you're going to see Dr. Greco soon. Talk to her about it!"

Then the patient sees another doctor, who says, "Well, you know, why don't we leave it up to Helen Greco to decide for you? I'll give you the prescription, I have some here, and if she says fine, then go on it."

But of everyone involved, no one asked her the most important question.

I said, "This is all well and good, but why do *you* want to take HRT?"

"I don't know!"

"Well, my patients know why they're taking HRT. Are you taking it for heart disease? Is it for osteoporosis, or vaginal dryness, or the texture of your skin?" She did not remember. Maybe it was for memory!

"Oh, I know, my doctor says it could help prevent heart and bone disease."

I said, "Fine. So now you want to stop HRT because of denser breasts."

The results of her bone densitometry test were normal.

You want to help prevent osteoporosis? It's exercise, weight bearing exercise, and calcium supplementation.

So now she's taking her weights out of the closet. She's going to work out with her weights, and we'll do another bone densitometry in a year or two to follow up.

If she's had a marked loss in this time period since she's been off hormones, then I would consider giving her something preventive, something in addition to what she's doing. If there's no real big loss, and she's doing well with what she's doing, why does she need to take a pill anyway?

So it's interesting. She then says, "Well, you're right, I don't want to just take stuff and put it in my body unless there is a good reason."

What's happening now in medicine is that we all want to prevent disease, so women are getting these pills thrown at them. They have to know why they are pre-scribed medications. Is it really doing any good, or would it be better to make a lifestyle change to help prevent these problems? Some women may need a combination of both.

Women should be responsible and ask questions!

13. Vitamin E, HRT, evening primrose, acupuncture, calcium and soy...

Who can make sense of all this?

Why are there so many options but so little information about them?

The trouble is, women have been put on the back burner when it comes to health research.

It wasn't until a few years ago that the United States National Institutes of Health launched a 628 million dollar Women's Health Initiative.

It will involve 27,500 women, and half will be randomly assigned to HRT and the other half to placebo. Researchers will follow the women for at least eight years comparing the rates of heart disease, breast cancer, osteoporosis and other ailments. Now, this won't be completed until the year 2005.

In the meantime, there is widespread use of plant sources of estrogen or estrogenic compounds. These include the phytoestrogens found in soybeans, ginseng and green tea.

What we know about alternative sources of estrogen such as these is mostly from other cultures. Some women naturally have a diet high in these foods, and have fewer menopausal symptoms than women in the United States, as well as a lower incidence of both heart disease and breast cancer. But there may be other factors operating as well.

You may take HRT. But it might be soybeans, ginseng and green tea for me!

It's amazing how much soy women are drinking. This is a big year for soy.

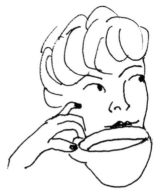

It is difficult to quantify how much estrogen is absorbed from these plant forms.

As for herbal alternatives, evening primrose is recommended for relief of everything from PMS symptoms to menopausal hot flashes. So is black cohosh, which is a plant root, but it is advised that women taking other hormonal drugs such as estrogen should not take it. A woman on HRT who takes black cohosh could end up with nausea, vomiting and headaches.*

Since these herbs aren't sold as medication that's regulated by the Federal Drug Administration, the labels may not contain any warnings and you could get in trouble.

Just because something is "natural" doesn't mean it's always safe for you, especially if you've been advised to avoid estrogen because of your medical condition. Your physician should be told if you are making any changes such as these in your diet.

*OB/GYN Special Edition, 1999, Vol 2, A Compendium of Educational Reviews, McMahon Publishing Group, N.Y., N.Y., page 52.

Other alternative therapies may include clonidine, an anti-hypertensive medication, or Bellergal. Either may help some women with hot flashes, night sweats and sleeplessness.

So there are choices, but it's important to know as much as you can about them. And talk to your physician.

14. Change of life. It can be a time when women don't know how to feel.

I think menopause is a difficult time for women because they're involved in a refocusing. Their bodies are changing, and things are changing all around them.

You have to redefine yourself, just like you did in adolescence!

A lot of phrases came about for this.

Menopause used to be called "change of life." And still sometimes you hear women talk about going through their "changes."

Many things do dramatically change when you hit this point in time.

I guess you feel you're not needed any more biologically, and there is a change in family roles.

It can be a time when women don't know how to feel.

It can be very difficult. Some women may become grandmothers and refocus and become caretakers again.

It's part of a time when priorities change, as well as levels of energy.

I don't know if everyone feels this, or I don't think they realize it. It's right in front of us.

Everything's changing and some women feel empty. Some may feel they have nothing to look forward to, or what they looked forward to before has changed.

Unless you've had hobbies before, but even then there's still a gap.

Now there's an empty nest, with children moving out and going ahead with their own lives.

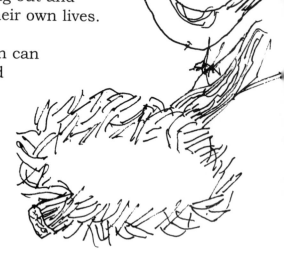

Sometimes a woman can feel really depressed about these things. There are whole arguments about depression in midlife, is it real or imagined? Sometimes a patient can just feel sad, and will ask for an anti-depressant or something for anxiety. That might be important. Even though there was no base-line problem to begin with, the stress of menopause may just tip you over.

Sometimes it all levels off, especially if time is taken to explain that what they're feeling is normal and may be helped with HRT. It is something to decide with your physician.

15. "Now what do I do?"

Someone called me today and we reviewed her FSH levels. That's the test I mentioned earlier that is used to determine estrogen levels. Her estrogen was very low. She was in menopause.

She said to me, "Now what do I do?"

I said, "Well, just do what you've been doing. Haven't you been exercising, and taking vitamins, calcium, and eating well?"

She's actually very knowledgeable.

She said, "Yes, I've been doing that, but what else can I do, what else can I expect, short-term, long-term?"

Again, in discussing any treatment, it is important to realize your own personal risk for cardiovascular disease, osteoporosis, and breast cancer.

It's all a very personal decision that is made in consultation with your physician.

As a woman reaches menopause and estrogen production stops, the skin on her face and all over her body can become dry. So I explain that you have to maintain the health of your skin more carefully now. Not just your face, but skin everywhere in your body is affected by the drop in estrogen, and that includes the vagina. Tissue there needs to be protected against getting thinner and becoming less flexible.

We take so many things for granted now.

At the time of the turn of the century, when women were wearing long dresses and corsets, and everything was so formal, just imagine how hard it was to talk about these things! That's why I think women were kept at home in their rooms when they didn't feel well. They drank teas and tonics and took vapors. None of this could be mentioned to their husbands, certainly, and perhaps only rarely even to a physician.

So I explain that you must moisturize the vagina as well. Most patients right away say, "Oh, of course!"

All kinds of products are now available over the counter including suppositories that contain vitamin E and aloe vera. Lubricants can also be very helpful. Estrogen in a cream form, as well as in the shape of a ring placed vaginally, can help restore the normal integrity of the vagina.

I want to say to these women, "You are not going to wake up turned to stone overnight!"

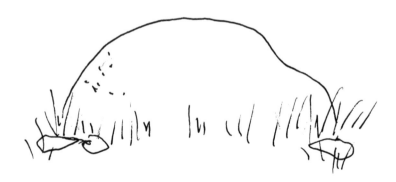

It's a gradual process. But you have to take care of your skin as you get older, and maintaining vaginal health is just as important.

16. "I'm done with menopause and if you mention it one more time I'll kill you!"

For some of my patients, like the one who said this, I think it's reassuring to know there are some real reasons for the strange changes in mood that can be experienced during this time of perimenopause and menopause.

So here are some facts about menopausal madness!

In fact:
Women in premenopausal years, that's ages 35-50, frequently show the effects of hormonal decline typical of these years with symptoms of premenstrual tension, irritability, mood lability, anxiety, depression, and migraines, also restless sleep, chronic fatigue, declining libido and, of course, irregular menstrual cycles.*

---

*Cooke DJ. A psychological study of the climacteric. In: Broome A, Wallace L, eds. *Psychology and genaecological problems*. London: Tavistock Publications. 1984; 243-265.
Dennestein L, Burrows GD, Hyman GJ, et al. Hormone therapy and affect. *Maturitas* 1979; 1:247-259.

In fact:

The declining levels of hormones during peri-menopause may also be connected with a higher incidence of depression and anxiety disorders. This can be explained because estrogen and progesterone have been shown directly to affect the neurotransmitters in the brain that regulate mood, appetite, sleep and pain perception.*

In fact:

After HRT for a 6-month period, 40% of the women experienced marked improvement in the categories of sleep disturbances, hot flashes, anxiety attacks, depression, as well as decreased short-term memory.**

In fact:

Estrogen and progesterone are known to alter the electrical and chemical features of the cells in the central nervous system, especially the hypothalamus. Changes in levels of these ovarian hormones influence specific central nervous system neurotransmitters that modulate mood, such as dopamine, norepinephrine, acetycholine and serotonin.*

*McEwen BS, Rhodes JC. Gonadal hormone regulation of MAO and other enzymes in hypothalamic areas. *Neuroendocrinol* 1983; 36: 235-238.
McEwen BS. Ovarian hormone action in the brain: Implications for the menopause. In Notelovitz M, Van Keep PA, eds. *The climacteric in perspective.* Lancester, England: MTP Press. 1976; 207-209.
McEwen BS. Basic research perspective: Ovarian hormone influence on the brain neurochemical function. In: Gise IH, ed. *Contemporary issues in obstetrics and gynecology: The premenstrual syndromes.* New York: Churchill-Livingstone. 1988: 21-33.
**Sarrel P. Ovarian steroids and the capacity to function at home and in the workplace. Presented at the North American Menopause Society Meeting (NAMS). New York, September 21-23, 1989.

In fact:
Objectively measured studies have been done of nocturnal hot flashes, and they confirm that they cause sleep waking episodes that can lead to chronic sleep deprivation and then to disturbances in mood (irritablity and depression), energy level, concentration, memory and overall mental well-being.*

In fact:
The word hysteria comes from the Greek word *hyster* which means womb. It was part of the every day language used by the early Greek physician Hippocrates, remembered for the Hippocratic oath which is still the code of ethics for the medical profession. He used the word hysteria to describe a disordered behavior exclusive to women related to the migration of the uterus. The adjective hysterical was quickly picked up by the men to explain to their satisfaction and glee why women seemed to them to behave more emotionally.

*Erlik Y, Tatryn IV, Meldrum DR, et al. Association of waking episodes with menopausal hot flushes. *JAMA* 1981; 245: 1741-1744.
Klaiber EL, Broverman DM, Bogel W, at al. Effects of estrogen therapy on plasma MAO activity and EEG driving responses of depressed women. *Am J Psychiatry* 1972; 128:42-48.
Thompson J, Oswald I. Effect of estrogen on the sleep, mood and anxiety of menopausal women. *Br Med J* 1977; 2:1217-1219.

17. "I Forgot !"

Uh oh! Look at this line I found in a book! I have to write it here for you.

"Recent studies suggest that estrogen decline at menopause may have a specific role in this process of declining cognitive function after the age of fifty."*

Oh boy, are we in trouble!

From studies it is felt that there is an overall clinical effect of estrogen on the enhancement of memory, short-term more than long-term, not visual memory, and verbal skills, as well as keeping the thinking process from deteriorating.**

This is interesting that when estrogen is in short supply, memory and thought processes may suffer!

A psychologist at Montreal's McGill University has studied the effects of estrogen therapy on women who have had their ovaries removed and produce very little estrogen on their own. She found that women who were given injections of estrogen were better at learning and recalling pairs of words than those in a group given a placebo. In the test it's very specific. It involves verbal tasks at which women tend to excel, but not visual

---

*Phillips SM, Sherwin BB. Effects of estrogen on memory function in surgically menopausal women. *Psychoneuroendocrinology* 1992: 17: 485-495.
**Lvine,VN. Estriol increases choline acetyltransferase activity in specific basal forebrain nuclei and projection area of female rats. *Exp Neurol* 1985; 89: 484-490.

memory.*

If I only had a brain!

So as you know, there is
a normal rise and fall of
estrogen throughout a
woman's menstrual cycle,
each month, which can
affect mental performance.*
In the McGill University
study, young women do
better on word-pair memory
tests during the phase of
their cycle when estrogen
and progesterone levels are
high than during menstruation
when hormone levels are low.

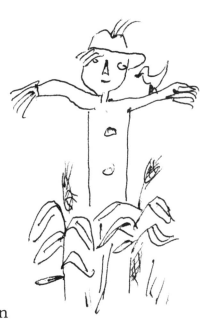

This doesn't mean women are less confident later in
their cycles. But it can explain minor changes that
some women notice where there's a little fogginess or
forgetfulness as women approach menopause. This can
be a direct result of low estrogen. The fog generally lifts
on its own, so the psychologist says, but hormone
replacement therapy may bring a break in the clouds.*

What's hard for some women is that they don't expect
this short-term memory loss to happen.

It can be very upsetting.

It may not be such a big deal, but it can start affecting
your daily living. You may have to write notes and leave

*Claudia Wallace, *Time Magazine,* June 26, 1995, "A Tonic for the Mind."

little messages everywhere.

I had a patient who was very upset. She said, "I can't remember the way I used to."

She is a dancer, and could learn a routine very quickly. She prided herself on picking up those steps right away. She can't now. That was scary for her.

There are a lot of changes with cognitive abilities, as well as some memory loss, that are occurring. A great fear arises for Alzheimer's disease.

In fact, evidence is accumulating showing that estrogen may reduce the risk of Alzheimer's disease.

Estrogen increases the production of acetylcholine, a brain chemical that is abnormally low in Alzheimer's patients. It may sensitize neural growth sites responsible for maintaining axon-dendrite or nerve cell connections in the brain.* More recent studies suggest estrogen effect is not global but specific, influencing neurons in the cerebral cortex, the hippocampus region which helps govern memory, and also the basal forebrain.**

These are the regions most affected in Alzheimer's disease which we know is more prevalent in aging women.

---

* Lvine,VN. Estriol increases choline acetyltransferase activity in specific basal forebrain nuclei and projection area of female rats. *Exp Neurol* 1985; 89: 484-490.

**Sohraabji F, Miranda RC, et al. Estrogen differentially regulates estrogen and nerve growth factor receptor MRNAs in adult sensory neurons. *J Neurosci* 1994; 14: 459-471.

In fact there were some small scale tests of estrogen with women who have mild to moderate Alzheimer's disease. These patients didn't know the month or year but could recall them after just three weeks on daily doses of hormones. They became more alert, ate and slept better, and showed improved social behavior.*

As you know, estrogen hasn't been approved for Alzheimer's disease, but as evidence builds, I think that this might be a good way to prevent memory loss in some women. Then it might be something to discuss with your physician.

---

*Claudia Wallace, *Time Magazine,* June 26, 1995, "A Tonic for the Mind."

18. Brie cheese.

"As far as I know, estrogen is made in fat cells. So I'll never get osteoporosis. I'll just keep eating brie cheese!"

Brie Cheese? No kidding?

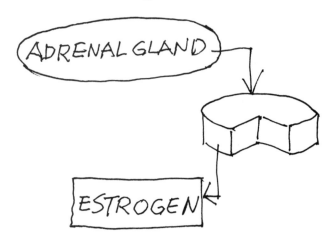

You know that throughout our lives women may produce estrogen from different sources.

During the reproductive years, estrogen is produced primarily by the ovaries.

When a woman is pregnant, there is an abundance of estrogen produced by the placenta.

But in menopause, there is no placenta and there are no functional ovaries, so where does the estrogen come from?

In menopause a very weak form of estrogen known as estrone is made in a woman's fatty or adipose tissue. There is a hormone called androstenedione that is produced by the adrenal glands located near the kidney. Androstenedione is converted in the fatty tissue into estrone. Heavier women produce much more estrone since they have more fatty tissue. That is what protects them from osteoporosis and keeps them from having hot flashes. It's also what puts them at risk for endometrial cancer.

Importantly, do you really know what obesity means besides just being overweight or heavy? It is the excessive storage of triglycerides in fatty or adipose tissue.

Did you know that throughout a woman's life, obesity increases threefold and reaches a plateau at approximately age 65?*

Estrogen or not, the brie's not worth it!

*Barrett-Connor E., Obesity, atherosclerosis, and coronary artery disease. *Ann Intern Med.* 1985; 103 :1010.

19. All about your bones.

Whereas life expectancy once exceeded menopause by only 10 years, we are now expected to be spending as much as a third of our lives beyond it. For that entire time, women will be without the hormones that sustained them during their earlier, reproductive years. One area of the body in particular that is protected by estrogen is the bones, and they are now at risk for becoming weakened and then fracturing.

But don't think of osteoporosis as a normal part of aging, and then ignore it. Do something about it!

Before menopause, estrogen allows a woman's bones to retain calcium and other minerals that help build bone strength. Estrogen is also needed to replace the bone loss that occurs in the natural process of the bone's tearing down and rebuilding itself in order to stay healthy.

Our peak bone mass is reached in our mid-thirties. But here are some alarming facts: During the first 10 years following menopause, women lose approximately 10% to 20% of bone mineral density. As a result, low bone mass density may be present in more than half of post-menopausal women.[*] Caucasian women by 80 years of age may have lost 50% of their skeletal mass.[**]

This is generally called Type I or Postmenopausal

[*]Genant Hk, Engelke K, Fuerst T, et. al. Noninvasive assessment of bone mineral and structure: state of the art. *J. Bone Min Pharm.* 1996: 11: 707-730.

[**]Riffee JM, Osteoporosis: Prevention and management. *Ann Pharm.* 1992; 32: 665-676.

Osteoporosis. There is also Type II which is related to long-term calcium deficiency, and this accounts for only very, very few of the fractures that occur in people over 70 years of age.

Currently more than 22 million women are at risk for osteoporosis, with an occurrence of over 1 million fractures annually. One out of every two women over age 50 will have an osteoporotic fracture in her lifetime and suffer one or more vertebral fractures as a result of osteoporosis.* The estimated numbers of women dying from complications of hip fractures alone is between 10% and 20%.**

But don't despair! Bone densitometry testing and preventive therapeutic treatments have been developed.

So you're not doomed to have broken bones if you take action!

Every woman who goes through menopause loses bone. A lot depends upon your peak bone mass prior to this time. If you start menopause with a lower bone mass, your bone mass density is already decreased.

Those women who are less at risk for osteoporosis have a higher bone mass density because they may be larger framed to begin with. Heavier women also make a certain amount of estrogen in their fatty tissue which will help prevent osteoporosis.

*National Institutes of Health, Osteoporosis and Related Bone Diseases - National Resource Center, Revised March, 1998, p. 1.
**Cooper C, Atkinson EJ, O'Fallon WM, Melton LJ III. The incidence of clinically diagnosed vertebral fractures: a population-based study in Rochester, Minnesota, 1985-1989. Bone Miner Res. 1992; 7:221-227.

Some risk factors relate to taking care of yourself.

If you're sedentary, a heavy smoker, a big caffeine or alcohol drinker, taking steroids or thyroid hormone, you're at risk. If there is a family history of osteoporosis, that should be considered as a risk factor, unless the condition was due to bad habits. These are things to discuss with a physician.

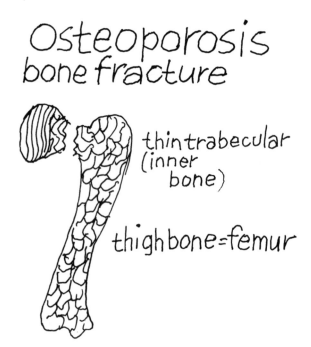

Osteoporosis
bone fracture

thin trabecular
(inner
    bone)

thigh bone=femur

20. You won't see a cave woman who has osteoporosis!

There was no problem of low bone mass density back then!

Even though they had no supplements to add calcium to their diets, no treadmills for weight bearing exercise, and as far as we know nobody was on hormone replacement therapy.

What made women so strong 5,000 years ago?

Let's start with the calcium. It was a very important component in the diet of early humans.

Calcium is the fifth most abundant element in the Earth's crust. Calcium is an important and essential building block of animals and plants. Our bones use up most of the calcium in our bodies, but what's left is very important.

We know calcium best from how it works in those amazing ways to get children into adulthood by building strong bones.

But here's what else calcium does: It helps nerves tell muscles when to contract thereby preventing cramps, it makes the impulse between nerves and the brain flow smoother, it aids in digestion by helping us produce saliva and enzymes, and it has a role in blood clotting to help heal wounds. A benefit just recently discovered, calcium seems to ease PMS!

Cave women had more calcium in their diets than anyone else in history!

That's why they probably didn't have much PMS. Otherwise cavemen would want to club them to death, and the evolution of women would have been gone.

Apparently the primitive hunter-gatherers consumed anywhere between 2000 to 3000 mg of calcium per day. Today, just 1500 mg a day is what's recommended for a woman in menopause.

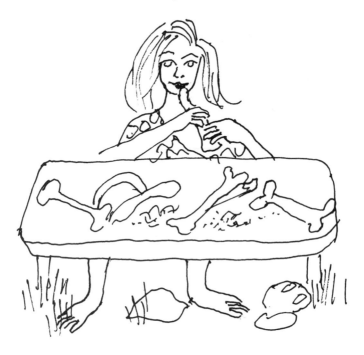

The human physiology adapted to this high intake of calcium, and developed ways to prevent against overdose and toxicity at those high levels. Our bodies today work pretty much the same way. But most women today do not obtain a sufficient amount of dietary calcium due to our reduced intake of foods that have high amounts of this element. We have failed since pre-history to evolve mechanisms for efficient calcium conservation.

Added to that, we don't have good net absorption efficiency of the element of calcium. It averages only 10% of the total calcium consumed. The kidney controls the preservation of calcium and regulates sodium, potassium, and protein. These can all get excreted by the kidneys and lost that way. The skin is also a regulator of these things. Our kidney calcium conservation is very poor, and our skin calcium loss is not regulated by the body at all. Added to that, these functions also deteriorate with age.

As for exercise, that could help strengthen our bones, too,but nothing today compares with the cave woman's workout of hauling whole mastodons into the kitchen and onto the barbecue spit.

The biggest difference, of course, is that while women reach peak bone mass in their mid-thirties, our earliest ancestors of course probably did not live to that age!

Even among our more recent ancestors, many women at the turn of the last century didn't live long enough to reach menopause.

As of the year 2000, 65,000,000 women will have reached menopause!

Many of them will be low in calcium, short on exercise, and lacking in hormones.

21. 86% of the people who have osteoporosis are not being treated at all!

Osteoporosis is a silent disease. As you know, there are two silent diseases that women have, and that would be cardiovascular disease and osteoporosis.

Just as you realize heart disease is often demonstrated by a heart attack because people cannot feel atherosclerosis, a fracture is usually the first demonstration that a person's bones have become dangerously fragile.

We currently can determine a person's probability for fracture in advance and offer preventive measures for most people who are at risk for developing osteoporosis. Of course the best thing is that parents, now armed with the facts about bone density, should make sure their children consume adequate amounts of calcium and vitamin D, stay physically active throughout childhood, and avoid smoking and alcohol so as to protect any bones that are at stake.

Now finding out about your bone mass density is important, especially if you are at high risk. All women 65 and older, regardless, should be tested.

An early test may save you from becoming at risk.

Do you know that 71% of women with osteoporosis don't know they have it!*

That's what makes osteoporosis a silent killer. There is no need today for that to be the case!

*Jane Brody, "Personal Health," New York Times, November 10, 1998.

What is a bone densitometry test?

Is it invasive? Does it hurt? Does it take long?

A bone densitometry test is not a regular x-ray, because a regular x-ray only shows bone loss after it is well advanced. The test that is recommended measures actual bone density in the spine, hip or wrist. It takes only a few minutes while you're lying down, and involves a very small amount of radiation. Other low radiation tests are also available, and some measure the bones of the forearm, finger, or heel, or others the spinal bone, or the knee.

The test results are based on a comparison of the bone density of a young adult before significant bone loss occurs. The results of the test are given in standard deviations (SD) from this norm. If the World Health Organization criteria, developed specifically for the spine, is extended to any skeletal region, women with a bone mass between 1 and 2.5 SD below the young adult mean is "osteopenic" which shows a shortage of bone mass. Anything at 2.5 SD or more below normal would would be called osteoporosis.*

What is very strange is that 86% of the people who have osteoporosis are not being treated at all!**

Estrogen replacement therapy is FDA-approved for treatment of osteoporosis and can decrease spinal and hip fracture by 50%. It can increase hip and spinal

*Lila A Wallis, MD. MACP, Anne Kasper , et al., Textbook of Women's Health, 1998, Lippincott-Raven, Philadelphia - New York, p.449.
**Jane Brody, "Personal Health,"New York Times, November 10, 1998.

bone density by approximately 2% per year.*

Alendronate is FDA-approved for both prevention and treatment of osteoporosis and can decrease spinal and hip fracture by 50%. It can increase hip and spinal density by about 2% per year.*

A new therapy is raloxifene, which prevents bone loss and may reduce the risk of spinal fracture 40% to 50%. It's a new class of drug called selective estrogen receptor modulators (SERM). It recently has been FDA-approved for the treatment of osteoporosis, and it also has a positive effect on LDL cholesterol.*

Another medication, calcitonin, may reduce spinal fractures by approximately 40% and increase spinal bone density by 1% - 2% per year. Its effect on the hip is still under review. It is administered as a nasal spray. It has been FDA-approved as a treatment for osteoporosis.*

They are all important tools, expecially since we now can determine so easily when therapy for osteoporosis is needed. Your physician can help you determine which treatment, if any, is necessary for you. In addition, physical therapy for osteoporosis may also be part of this regimen.

If women take care of themselves and take advantage of what medical technology and knowledge have to offer, we can silence that silent killer, osteoporosis!

*Ob/Gyn Special Edition, 1999, Vol 2, A Compendium of Educational Reviews, McMahon Publishing Group,NY, NY, page 24.

22. Now there's a new calcium supplement that tastes like a chewy caramel.

I want to go back to the cave women again, their diet, and how they consumed so much more calcium than we do. Today a woman's body still works on the need for the large amount of calcium they were used to.

If a woman today cannot tolerate dairy products, there are certain vegetables that are good sources of calcium. These would include dark green leafy vegetables such as collards, broccoli or bok choy, and tofu, salmon, and sardines with bones. There also are many fortified foods.

So the cave women probably ate a lot of green vegetables, and bones. They weren't allowed to eat the good stuff, so they got their calcium from bones.

Whatever was going on, they were doing better than our teenagers. Look at teenagers! They're supposed to be getting a lot of calcium so they may go into the next phase of life with the maximum bone mass.

Now where are they getting their calcium from?

French fries and sodas?

Sometimes a supplement is required. A chewable supplement is good because disintegration of a pill can be a problem. Calcium carbonate is an excellent source of calcium. It's highly bio-available and it's well absorbed by everyone including those who lack gastric acid in their stomach, so long as it is consumed with food.

Absorbability from most of the calcium supplements varies little. It's very important that a person who takes calcium takes one that she can tolerate well without difficulty. So if one calcium supplement is intolerant, then another would be fine, such as calcium citrate.

The best way for a calcium supplement to be absorbed is in divided doses with a meal. In order to have good absorption of calcium you need vitamin D supplementation to help assist in this, approximately 400-800 international units per day.

Now what I also wanted to mention very importantly is that the calcium requirement of anywhere from 1200 to 1500 mg each day is for those who consume a typical American diet. There are several dietary components which can change calcium requirement quite a bit, such as sodium (salt) and protein. These lead to increased calcium loss from the kidneys.

So women with low intakes of both nutrients, sodium and protein, have a calcium requirement that's much lower. They lose less calcium. Whereas women who take in more sodium and protein than the national average have requirements as high as 2000 mg a day.

Now there's a calcium supplement in a chewy caramel. Yummy!

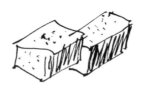

23. Calcium, HRT and your bones.

Calcium and vitamin D supplementation can decrease spinal fracture 10% - 15% per year, decrease hip fracture 25% per year, and increase hip bone density 1% per year.* Now that is quite impressive!

I don't think women realize how important it is to maintain their bone mass, importantly before menopause, and more importantly once they've reached menopause.

I mentioned briefly before how bone is constantly tearing down and building up to stay strong and healthy. I'd like to explain this a little more now.

In a healthy adult, approximately 6% to 10% of skeleton is turned over each year in a process called skeletal bone remodeling.** It occurs every day, and it's involved with two parts that make up the bone: osteoclasts and osteoblasts. Osteoclasts break down, and osteoblasts build up. The bone is changing constantly. There's constant bone remodeling in which microscopic volumes of bone are removed by osteoclastic resorption, and then the resultant cavities are filled in by osteoblastic deposition of new bone.

Now very interestingly, estrogen treats the underlying physiology of bone loss. It promotes a decrease in bone breakdown.

*OB/GYN Special Edition, 1999, Vol 2, A Compendium of Educational Reviews, McMahon Publishing Group, NY, NY, page 52.
**Lila A Wallis, MD. MACP, Anne Kasper, et.al., Textbook of Women's Health, 1998, Lippincott-Raven, Philadelphia - New York, p. 447.

Estrogen replacement therapy can help prevent the 15% loss of bone that occurs at menopause, at least as long as estrogen is being taken in an adequate dose and is continued.

In order for bone to regenerate, it requires an appropriate amount of calcium as well as vitamin D. So osteoporosis involves a number of conditions, it's multifactorial, in which calcium deficiency plays the major role. That's why women more than ever are encouraged to maintain and supplement their diet. They're supposed to supplement to begin with, which no one does, then in menopause it's more than necessary.

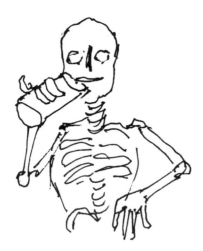

There are genetic factors and metabolic regulations that also affect calcium. It can be impacted by thyroid and parathyroid function, as well as extraneous factors such as diet and of course the lack of weight bearing exercise. Prior falls may also affect osteoporosis, as well as inactivity.

The greatest impact in a woman's life span for calcium supplementation in terms of reducing fracture actually occurs before she reaches peak bone mass, meaning in her teenage years. If you start off with greater bone mass before you go into menopause, you're ahead of the game.

A very good way to prevent osteoporosis is not only

adequate amounts of calcium and vitamin D in the daily diet but...dancing, a walk at lunch break, or how about tai chi! Exercise that is weight-bearing, which includes balancing and strengthening, at least 30 minutes a day, is not only good for the bones, but is also good for the soul.

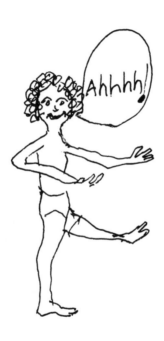

24. Heart Disease.

There are other events that may occur from this natural process we call menopause. One long term complication would be heart disease.

Heart disease is the leading cause of death among women, claiming more lives than cancers of the breast, cervix, uterus, and ovary combined.

Even though heart attacks have been thought of as a male disease, more women die of cardiovascular disease each year than men do. It is the leading cause of death among women over 50.

A heart attack manifests itself differently in a woman than in a man. It may feel more like a passing chest pain, or even stomach pain. If you suspect it's a heart problem, you must speak up about that silent killer!

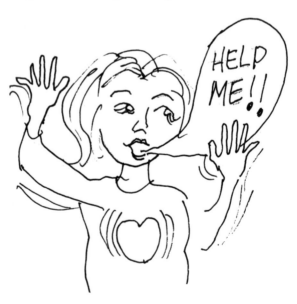

Although there is still some uncertainty, it seems probable that the loss of estrogen after menopause increases a woman's risk of developing heart disease. For one thing, estrogen helps keep cholesterol levels in check.*

By the age of 85, 1 in 2 women will have heart disease!**

Although 1 in 26 women will die of breast cancer, almost 1 in 2 will die of cardiovascular disease.**

1 in 10 women ages 45 to 64 has some form of cardiovascular disease.**

Every year since 1984, cardiovascular disease has claimed the lives of more women than men.**

It's heart disease that gets us in the end!

But coronary heart disease is largely a preventable problem!

There are many factors that are not necessarily genetic that put a woman at risk for heart disease. These can be diagnosed, and in many cases corrected.

That's true for everything from high cholesterol to high blood pressure, and from diabetes to obesity.

All women over 50 should have their cholesterol checked.

* The Female Patient, Vol. 24, May 1999, p. 47.
** Issues in Women's Health/Media Kit, 1999, p.5.

Regarding cholesterol, the HDL, or High Density Lipoprotein, has a positive role. It takes cholesterol from the blood to the liver, where it is broken down and disposed of. The LDL or Low Density Lipoprotein, has a negative function. It takes cholesterol into the body's arteries where it causes them to clog.

Another type of fat to watch for is triglycerides.

The numbers below show normal or desirable levels for cholesterol and triglycerides. Be aware that there is individual laboratory variability.

	Level (mg/dl)
Total cholesterol	< 200
HDL -cholesterol	> 35-60
LDL-cholesterol	< 130
Triglycerides	< 200

Don't just accept something is not good and then not do anything about it!

Blood cholesterol levels have a lot to do with whether or not your heart stays healthy.

Some other risk factors for cardiovascular disease are genetic. You would know about this if your father or mother had a history of heart disease. It's worse if your mother had heart disease in her 40's, and it's not very good if your father died of a heart attack at 50. But sometimes their illnesses are related to lifestyles, and that would not affect you in the same way.

*Cholesterol and Your Heart, American Heart Association,1993,pp.10-13.

Hypertension or high blood pressure can put a person at risk for heart disease. If there is a lot of plaque in arteries it takes a higher pressure to push the blood through. Stress can create high blood pressure as well.

Just as there are medications for problematic high cholesterol that can't be controlled by diet and exercise alone, there is medication for hypertension, too.

Diabetes and obesity can also put you at risk for heart disease. They can and should be treated!

Did you realize that obesity is associated with 4 major risk factors for hardening of the arteries?

1. Diabetes
2. Hypertension
3. Elevated cholesterol
4. Elevated tryglicerides

The combination of any one of these risk factors with obesity significantly increases the risk of heart disease, cerebrovascular disease, and death.*

*Byyny RL, Speroff L. A Clinical Guide for the Care of Older Women: Primary and Preventive Care (2nd ed). Baltimore, Md: Williams & Wilkins; 1996.

25. Heart disease: A preventable problem.

The fear regarding heart disease is that it's a silent killer.

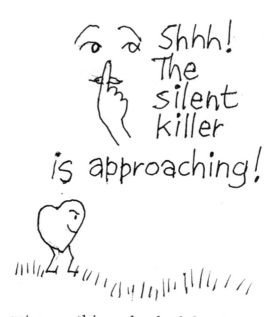

Shhh! The silent killer is approaching!

Many women get everything checked for their hearts, but don't listen, and somehow are not treated!

You can help your heart in many ways!

After menopause this is very important because the heart is no longer protected by estrogen.

Many women feel they can take care of their hearts themselves, and it's true. The health of your heart is one thing, it's a muscle. You can exercise it like you strengthen other muscles in your body, like your arms and legs. Aerobic exercise strengthens the heart.

You can take care of the blood going through your

heart by eating well and avoiding fatty foods. A healthful diet and good nutrition can help keep your LDL cholesterol down and that helps keep arteries unclogged.

Some women have a genetic predisposition for high cholesterol, and that has to be managed, too. Just because it's genetic doesn't mean it's normal. Lots of women say, "My mother had it, it's in our genes." So what! Do you just leave it alone? No. You have to do something about it!

Obesity, excessive alcohol consumption, and cigarette smoking put a person at risk, and so does a sedentary lifestyle.

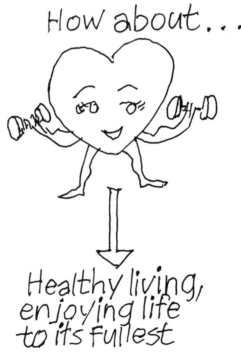

How about...

Healthy living, enjoying life to its fullest

So why not do something good for your heart instead?

26. Heart disease: What the tests show.

Now we know that cardiovascular disease accounts for nearly 375,000 deaths in women each year.*

Pretty frightening!

When we talk about heart disease, that includes heart attacks, heart failure, high blood pressure, and clogged arteries.

Ongoing studies are being done for menopausal women regarding the impact of low estrogen on heart disease.

The Postmenopausal Estrogen/Progestin Interventions (PEPI) Trial reported in November, 1994, that hormone replacement regimens produced significant increases in the levels of HDL or good cholesterol. With everything we know, that meant HRT would strongly protect women against coronary disease.

Another study went further. Instead of just showing how HRT affected cholesterol levels in the blood, it followed women taking HRT to see if in fact there was a change in the actual incidence of cardiac events.

The earliest results of the Heart and Estrogen/Progestin Replacement Study (HERS) were published in August, 1998, and boy was everyone surprised.

What do you think the HERS study showed us about HRT and heart disease in postmenopausal women?

*National Center for Health Statistics; Monthly Vital Statistics Report. 1995; 45 (11) Supp 2.

HERS found that there was no significant difference in the number of coronary heart disease events, or deaths from them, for women who already had established heart disease.The trial included 2,763 postmenopausal women with cardiovascular disease.*

So now we have to remind women that although HRT can reduce as much as half the risk for heart disease, it is only if they have healthy hearts to begin with!

With established heart disease, it is not so. We now know that the risk of a blood clot is increased the first two years that you put a patient with heart disease on hormones. Although if she is already on HRT for 4 years and is doing well, it could be appropriate for her to be on it.* A decision such as this must be made by a patient in consultation with her physician.

Now the next giant step in testing for women is the Women's Health Initiative involving 27,500 women. This will be completed in the year 2005. Heart disease as well as osteoporosis will be studied, as they relate to HRT and also diet.

We can't wait for the results of that!

Not everyone is so sure that HRT is the answer for all women concerned about heart disease. Exercise and good nutrition are a must. And no smoking!

I think it's unfair for women to feel they have to take

*Hulley Stephen, Grady Deborah, Bush Trudy,et al. Randomized Trial of Estrogen Plus Progestin for Secondary Prevention of Coronary Heart Disease in Postmenopausal Women. *JAMA*, August 19, 1998, Volume 280: 605-613.

hormones otherwise they're doomed. I think HRT can be quite helpful, but more importantly it's your attitude and lifestyle that makes a difference. Understanding the changes your body is going through will also help you.

27. HRT and breast cancer.

It's heart disease which is the silent killer of women, and with osteoporosis they're the two main problems and causes of morbidity and mortality to women.

But all we worry about is breast cancer!

We have a tremendous fear of losing what I think some women feel is their femaleness because they can see this when they look in the mirror. They see the loss or change in their breasts, and the limitation they feel that may be placed upon them if they have breast cancer.

Breast cancer is the No. 1 occurring cancer in American women, with more than 175,000 new cases reported every year.* It is second only to lung cancer as a cause of death from cancer in U.S. women, so there are fewer deaths from breast cancer than from lung cancer.

43,300 women die of breast cancer a year!*

But as many as 70% of women with breast cancer have no family history.

In fact, studies exploring the possible cause-and-effect relationship between estrogen replacement therapy and breast cancer generally are reassuring.

A comprehensive analysis of more than 90% of the

*American Cancer Society, Cancer Facts and Figures - 1998.

original global data on breast cancer and estrogen/hormone therapy was conducted in 1997 by the Collaborative Group on Hormonal Factors in Breast Cancer. The group concluded that the use of estrogen/hormone therapy for about 13 years would result in one extra breast cancer being diagnosed per 100 women.*

But for women who have been on HRT for 10 or more years, there is still some uncertainty. So that's the next question.

Women will ask, "What should I do?"

I will advise them. "Your risk of breast cancer does increase as you age. Whether you're taking hormones or not, the risk is there." It is important to consult with your physician, someone who has examined you and is fully aware of your medical and family history.

Estrogen replacement therapy will promote the growth of breast cancer, but will usually not initiate it at the low doses that are classically used. So why should you stop estrogen after 5 or 10 years? All the benefits you have gained from HRT will stop, and all the untoward effects of menopause will return!

As you start to age you worry about, well, all these cancers, and then you start looking at what you're taking and the constant contradiction in the media. If you weren't confused before, you sure could be now!

*Collaborative Group on Hormonal Factors in Breast Cancer. Breast cancer and hormone replacement therapy: collaborative reanalysis of data from epidemiological studies of 52,705 women with breast cancer and 108,411 women without breast cancer. *Lancet.*, 1997:350:1047-1059.

I have patients who take all this in stride, in a good spirit. They do understand all the fuss, but HRT is an essential part of their lives and well being. Many will say without reservation, "I'll take hormones until the day I die."

Although in some studies hormone therapy appears slightly to increase the diagnosis of breast cancer, hormone therapy use is also associated with decreased mortality from breast cancer.*

Women who are on HRT are followed very closely. There's earlier diagnosis of breast cancer in HRT users, as well as greater survival rate. Current users are associated with lower frequency of late stage disease. In general, HRT users develop better differentiated tumors.*

Regular breast examination by a health care provider and monthly self-examination are recommended for all women.

*Bergkvist L, Adami H-O, Persson I, et al. Prognosis after breast cancer diagnosis in women exposed to estrogen and estrogen-progestogen replacement therapy. *Am J Epidemiol.*. 1989;130:221-228.
Hunt K, Vessey M, McPherson K. Mortality in a cohort of long-term users of hormone replacement therapy: an updated analysis. *Br J Obstet Gynecol.*. 1990;97:1080-1086.
Strickland DM, Gambrell RD Jr, Butzin CA, et al . The relationship between breast cancer survival and prior postmenopausal estrogen use. *Obstet Gynecol.* 1992; 80:400-404.
Colditz GA, Hankinson SE, Hunter DJ, et al. The use of estrogen and progestins and the risk of breast cancer in postmenopaual women. *N Engl J Med.* 1995; 332:1589-1593.
Willis DB, Calle EE, Miracle-McMahill HL, Heath CW Jr. Estrogen replacement therapy and risk of fatal breast cancer in a prospective cohort of postmenopausal women in the United States. *Cancer Causes Control.* 1996; 7:449-457.
Grodstein F, Stampfer MJ, Colditz GA, et al.. Postmenopausal hormone therapy and mortality. *N Engl J Med.* 1997; 336:1769-1775.

If you feel a breast mass at any time, you must consult a physician! Even if the mammogram is normal!

Did you know that mammograms have a false negative rate of 10%? This means that 10% of the time if a mammogram is normal, it really may not be!

A baseline mammogram is recommended at age 35, unless there's a family history to warrant it sooner.

Women between the ages of 40 to 49 should have a mammogram every 1 to 2 years. Women over 50 should have a mammogram each year, even if everything seems fine, regardless of whether or not they're taking HRT.

The importance of early detection and diagnosis of breast cancer cannot be emphasized enough.

When we say 1 in 8 women in America develops breast cancer during her lifetime, that is 12.5% of the female population!*

The best way to alter the natural course of the disease is to take advantage of the opportunity for early discovery and diagnosis.

*SEER Cancer Statistics Review 1973-1993. Miller et al., eds. National Cancer Institute, 1997.

28. Has anyone checked your breasts lately? It should be you!

I have patients who come and will say, "Oh, I just had my mammogram, no need to examine my breasts."

I will respond, "That means nothing in terms of checking your breasts yourself. No one knows your breasts better than you!"

Very importantly, not all palpable masses of the breast can be seen by mammograms.

If you're young, or just have very dense or fibrocystic breasts, a breast sonogram may also be in order.

You may be able to feel a mass, but it's not well visualized.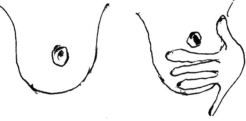

That's why any new palpable mass, even if not seen by a mammogram may require a biopsy. You must consult with your physician and perhaps even get a second, or third, opinion if there is any doubt.

A mammogram is still very important, because finding a tumor early is the best chance to treat it. The value of a mammogram is that it is able to identify breast abnormalities that may be cancerous at an early stage before physical symptoms develop.

Most doctors may feel a breast mass when it is 1cm in size or larger. But mammograms may demonstrate fine irregularities in breast cancers months to even years prior to their growing to a size that can be physically appreciated.

Women who are taking HRT are usually the most vigilant about checking their breasts. They're usually more involved with their care and their health.

If you feel there's something wrong, don't wait, call your doctor. How would they know if you don't call?

It's not rare to have breast cancer anymore, you know, so beware.

29. Get to know your breasts!

When a woman is taking hormones, you can tell, even after several weeks, there's a change in breast tissue. Hormones may make the breast denser, similar to a young breast.

The mammary gland, or breast, consists of 20% glandular tissue, and 80% fibrous connective tissue and fat.

The fibrous tissue is in the entire surface of the breast and also connects the tissue throughout. After menopause this tissue becomes less dense, and at the same time the amount of fat increases, just as it does elsewhere in the body. The lobes in the glandular tissue are like bunches of grapes, and after menopause they get smaller.

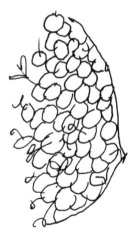

Altogether after menopause, without estrogen, a women's breasts aren't as firm. There's more fat, the fat isn't held up very well anymore, so the breasts sag.

Fat responds to aging, and everything is replaced by fat unless you exercise. And you're not going to exercise your breasts unless you're a topless dancer!

When you go on hormones, your fibrous tissue is not doing what a menopausal woman's should.

When some women go on hormones, they're so happy

because their breasts are so nice and full.

Others may not realize there's a difference that comes from being on hormones.

For all women, it's important that they get to know their own breasts!

I don't know your breasts like you know your breasts.

So I say over and over and over, "Check your breasts!"

The monthly self breast exam, as well as a physical exam by a physician, and mammography, are complementary procedures and they must be considered together.

A negative mammogram does not rule out breast cancer!

Women are very defensive about something happening to their breasts, as if they don't want to know. But sometimes they can know instinctively, it's their own body.

Many women are so unsure, or rather so afraid, they don't even say anything to their physician.

You know your breasts the best. You have to confide in your doctor.

Don't think it's all in your head!

30. Wrinkle.

I have a patient who is 80 years old, and she is in wonderful health, very lively, but the last time she came to see me, was she upset!

"Look at my wrinkles, I just got these wrinkles three months ago!"

Now she wants to start hormone replacement therapy, at age 80!

The process of wrinkling has to do with loss of dermal collagen, and it shows a 30% decline in the first 10 postmenopausal years, and that results in loss of skin thickness and elasticity.*

The collagen is a sort of gelatinous substance and in the body it is found in connective tissue, bone and cartilage. With the loss of collagen comes many other manifestations of what we think of as aging including vaginal mucosal atrophy, vascular fragility and urinary stress incontinence.

In what was considered a landmark study in 1983 in Great Britain, menopausal women were given estrogen and compared to subjects not taking hormones. Among the treated women, the mean collagen concentration was about 33% higher than those without treatment.*

Loss of collagen correlates well with loss of bone density, which also shows up to a 20% reduction in the first postmenopausal decade. In fact, the loss of dermal

*Ob.Gyn. News, May 1, 1999, p. 18.

collagen can be used to predict osteoporotic fracture as patients with the lowest collagen content have the highest risk of osteoporotic fracture.*

So any approach to hormone replacement therapy is likely to have some positive effect on the skin.

I'm not sure for 80 year olds, but since that's her only problem, she shouldn't get any more wrinkles having to worry about it.

*Ob.Gyn. News, May 1, 1999, P. 18.

31. It may not be menopause.

The thyroid is a very busy organ and it may slow down with aging.

Thyroid hormone is another widely prescribed medication for women in America.

A woman may have a decrease in her thyroid function at about the same time as her estrogen levels are starting to fluctuate.

If the thyroid isn't producing any hormones, it will send a signal to the hypothalamus, like the signals the ovary would send when there's a lack of estrogen. It will say to the hypothalamus, "Come on and put out some more of that releasing hormone, and make the pituitary try to put out more of the thyroid stimulating hormone." This can cause symptoms that are similar to hot flashes.

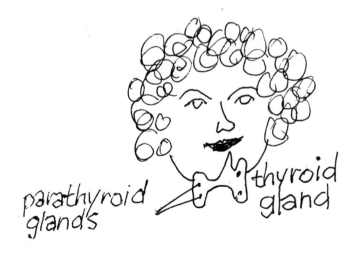

parathyroid
glands

thyroid
gland

That's why I make sure there's no thyroid disease, because it can mimic menopause. Some of these shared symptoms include heat intolerance, fatigue and mood swings.

The thyroid is involved in the remodeling of bone. The parathyroid glands are right around the thyroid, producing a hormone that works on the kidney to help preserve calcium.

A woman can also experience muscle aches, general body stiffness, hair loss and loss of skin tone. You have to be careful that there's no underlying medical condition such as thyroid disease, or arthritis. A physician should examine you. Do not just assume that some of your symptoms are related to the "normal" aging process.

This is a time when there are a lot of things to look out for.

You know what, I ask women if they've had their thyroid checked and they say, "Oh, my internist did a full checkup and blood work."

What does that mean exactly? And I ask,"Which blood tests?" They don't know!

Women should be empowered with information and know what to ask for from their physicians.

32. The vaginal garden.

I was speaking to a woman who was having a problem with vaginal infections, and I began talking about the vaginal ecosystem.

She said, "Why, it sounds as if you're talking about a garden!"

I don't remember thinking about it that way, but there is a balance that must be maintained in order for the vagina to be healthy. There's actually a pH balance, and the normal vagina is acidic and is very resistant to infections for that reason. There are a number of variables that influence the bacterial flora, as it's called, of the vagina.

These variables include the naturally acidic pH, oxygen, nutritional elements, moisture, temperature, and, with all that, competition among organisms for adherence sites to the vagina. It could be like a garden, I guess, maybe a shade garden.

One important element is glycogen, a starch-like substance that gets converted to sugar, or glucose, by bacterial enzymes. These same enzymes then ferment it to lactic acid. It's something like winemaking. That makes the proper pH balance which for a woman in her reproductive years is 3.8 to 4.5, a little too acidic for a vineyard, but that's what makes us able to resist infections.

Now when estrogen levels decrease in menopause, there is no stimulation for the production and deposition of this glycogen into the vaginal and cervical cells. Since there's less glycogen, there is less glucose or sugar available for conversion to lactic acid and thereby the vagina becomes less acidic, more basic. This makes a woman much more susceptible to vaginal infection.

When the acid level of the vagina is lower, it allows other bacteria that normally aren't there to colonize, like gastrointestinal bacteria. At the same time, certain species of lactobacilli which are normally present are missing. Lactobacilli are important in the production of hydrogen peroxide. This helps the vaginal flora's ability to resist infection.

This is similar to problems that can develop when a person is on antibiotic therapy or from douching excessively. Both can disturb the vaginal pH and then predispose to the creation of vaginal infection.

The vagina becomes infected, and the vulva and external urethra, which is where we void from, develop a type of inflammatory reaction causing the tissue to become inflamed. It can become irritated thereby creating a virulent type of discharge.

You can see why someone can become predisposed to urinary tract infections at this time. Vaginal intercourse can aggravate these types of changes that go on, and that's why there could be severe discomfort and bleeding.

If you do have bleeding during intercourse, do not assume it is a normal part of menopause. You must be examined by a physician.

I feel that if you keep the vagina moist, even though the pH of the vagina is changed, that would help maintain vaginal health.

This brings me to the topic of vaginal moisturizers.

Yes, there's a lack of estrogen, and if left unattended it really can get to a severe degree of inflammatory changes as I've just mentioned. If you try to maintain normal vaginal health with moisturizers, along with good nutrition, exercise, and good hygiene, of course, it helps maintain vaginal health as much as possible.

I recommend moisturizers with aloe vera and vitamin E, which is good at any point from perimenopause on. A woman may not even be sexually active, but just as a matter of prevention.

You have to pay attention and take care of these things.

33. Tending the vaginal garden.

I know a lot of women are hesitant taking HRT especially for vaginal dryness!

They're really wishy washy about estrogen. They feel like they're doing well, they have gotten past the hot flashes, and are not having mood swings, "But you know that dryness is a problem" is what they'll say.

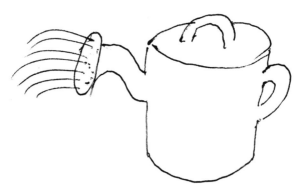

So I may recommend a vaginal lubricant or suppository. But then they might say, "You know intercourse is still uncomfortable."

At times difficulties can occur with vaginal atrophy because of the changes in the vagina from lack of estrogen. The tissue of the vaginal lining becomes thinner and less flexible, and the vagina itself may become shorter and narrower. At times there can also be problems because the vaginal walls may actually agglutinate or stick together, thereby making vaginal intercourse quite painful or nearly impossible.

Then something more than a vaginal moisturizer is needed. I'll recommend local estrogen cream once a week or an estrogen ring that is placed in the vagina. Estrogen used in this manner works mainly in the vagina, and at low doses is not absorbed into the system. This means it does not affect your heart, bones, breasts or uterus.

But should there be extreme vaginal shrinkage, vaginal dilators can be used to distend the vagina.

Loss of estrogen can also be related to incontinence with portions of the bladder walls and urinary tract becoming thinner and more fragile. They can thereby be prone to trauma and infection during vaginal intercourse.

There are, as you can see, some very personal problems that can arise at this time. I try to make sure my patients know what they can do to protect themselves.

34. Sex.

A patient of mine was reading a magazine article called something like "Making Lovemaking Last - How to Keep the Sizzle in Your Sex Life after Menopause."*

I said, "That looks interesting, quality sex."

She said, "I'll brush up on the quality, just let me have some!"

Sex is always mentioned when the topic of menopause comes around.

It comes down to this: It's a time in a woman's life when she could very well have the same interest she always had in having sex, or she could have less interest, or even more. Different studies say different things, that maybe there's a loss of desire, but from what I can tell, it depends on what each woman is feeling.

I think this is a time to enjoy, and have fun. Yeah, have fun! The kids are out, no one's home, you're not going to get pregnant.

Women can lose interest in sex because they lack not just estrogen, but also testosterone, a male type of hormone that is produced less by the ovaries after menopause. It's involved in keeping us interested in sex, also known as libido.

Another reason is: women aren't meant to have sex

*The American College of Obstetricians and Gynecologists, "Guide to Managing Menopause," Spring/Summer, 1999.

after menopause! Since the beginning of time, once you were too old to procreate, no more sex!

But sexual function is important for women regardless of age. Testosterone is beginning to be included in hormone replacement regimens. Early tests show it can make women feel better, and improve libido.

Despite anything nature intended for us, women after menopause are on the whole still very busy sexually.

In speaking of sex as part of a normal healthy life, I have to mention a serious health risk that concerns all of us today, and that is transmission of the AIDS virus. We should all still have fun, but we have to be careful, regardless of our age or our partner. Safe sex is still an issue.

35. And what exactly is sex?

Sex is all about bringing pleasure to yourself.

Sexual activity affects your body directly, it makes you feel good, it excites you and then relaxes you, and it adds to your health and well being.

There are different kinds of sexual experiences, either with a partner, pleasing each other, or just by pleasing yourself.

There are technically different phases your body experiences during sex, and both physiology and emotion are interwoven throughout. I will explain them.

In the first phase a person starts to feel a sense of desire and begins to have thoughts or images relating to sexual activity. This feeling makes us receptive to stimulation and excitement.

As these feelings intensify, our bodies begin to respond and then physiological changes occur that relate to sexual arousal. In this stage of excitement a woman's body starts to react, vaginal lubrication occurs, and the vaginal tissue becomes infused with blood and expands significantly. The clitoris, located above the vaginal opening, becomes highly sensitive, protruding, while internally the uterus elevates within the pelvis. The nipples of the breast become enlarged and erect throughout this phase. As stimulation and excitement progress, heart rate, breathing and blood pressure increase.

The release from this plateau of stimulation is called an

orgasm. This experience of overwhelming pleasure is derived from involuntary rhythmic muscular contractions involving the uterus, vagina and rectum, and it is accompanied by a release of muscular tension throughout the body. The respiratory rate, heart rate and blood pressure remain high, and this may last from between 3 to 60 seconds.

The final phase is the resolution phase, which brings us a general feeling of well-being, comfort and calmness. Physiologically, everything returns to its normal state.

We all experience the pleasures of sex differently, and these changes that occur during sex will often vary among us.

Everyone I think has different areas or spots that please them during sex. We may want to communicate this to our partner and that may be an important part of feeling satisfied. Some women may want to touch themselves while they are having sex or vaginal intercourse, and that's okay, too. Satisfying yourself when you are alone is also a part of natural good health.

It's important to relax so you can help your body enjoy itself. Aside from making babies, that's what sex is for. It's to please yourself.

36. A patient should find a doctor she can talk to and who will listen to her.

When a woman starts this time called menopause, a lot of changes happen to her body that she may not expect.

It's a time when your weight may change, which could be related to lifestyle, when you're exercising less, or eating more. In fact, your metabolism does change, it slows down, so it's important to be careful of what you eat, maybe skip a chocolate here or there. Try to take up exercise a little more seriously, because it's even more important at this time in your life.

Even so, no matter what you do, all of a sudden you find your summer shorts have shrunk over the winter, your shape's changed a bit, and a favorite sweater doesn't fit. You have to buy new bras, since the size of your breasts has changed, and new shoes, because your feet are different!

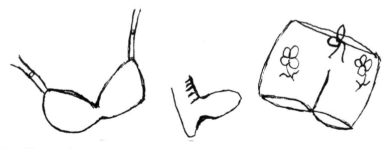

Really, a lot is going on.

Some women may need to have estrogen replaced.

Other women compensate for that loss of estrogen with changes in lifestyle, with healthful diets and weight bearing exercise, as well as maybe new hobbies.

Whenever I speak to a patient, I ask her questions about herself.

Just listening helps me get a better picture of her life and attitude, her level of happiness or stress. All this may affect her health.

A patient should find a doctor she can talk to and who will listen to her.

In the "olden" days, a patient would see a doctor only if she was not feeling well, when something was wrong.

Nowadays, with regular check ups, wellness visits, they're sometimes called, a woman can come in even when she's fine, and tell me she's just feeling well. We will plan her health care together. This is called preventive medicine.

37. What can go wrong: Cancer in women.

There are a lot of women usually going about their business and some of them may have cancer. Not often, but enough.

Cancer remains the second leading cause of death among adult women, the leading cause being heart disease.

1999 Cancer Estimates - U.S.*

Type		New Cases		Deaths
Breast	#1	175,000	#2	43,300
Lung		77,600	#1	68,000
Colorectal		67,000	#3	28,800
Uterus		37,400		6,400
Ovary		25,200		14,500
Urinary system		28,100		8,900
Non-Hodgkin's lymphomas		24,200		12,300
Melanoma of skin		18,400		2,700
Bladder		15,100		4,000
Pancreas		14,600		14,700**
Leukemia		13,400		9,700
Cervix		12,800		4,800
Oral		9,800		2,700
Vaginal and other genital		2,300		600

*Reprinted by the permission of the American Cancer Society, Inc.

**Note: Due to the high mortality of this form of cancer, deaths may exceed the incidence of new cases in any given year.

38. Tests to take, guidelines to follow.

These guidelines are an essential part of being in charge of your health now. Follow them, and be well. And always consult with your physician for any additional testing.

Breast Exam

Mammogram	Baseline at age 35*
	Every 1 to 2 years ages 40-49
	Yearly 50 and over
Self Exam	Monthly for all women
Pelvic Exam	Yearly for all women
Pap smear	Yearly for all women**
Blood pressure	Yearly for all women*
Blood Work	Every 2 to 3 years for women starting at
cbc, cholesterol,	age 40*
thyroid, and blood	
sugar	
EKG	Yearly for all women*
Rectal Exam	Yearly for all women age 40 and over*
Stool for occult	Yearly starting at age 40*
blood test	
Sigmoidoscopy	Every 3 to 5 years at age 50
Colonoscopy	Every 10 years after age 50*
Bone densitometry	At menopause or by age 65*
Urinalysis	Yearly after age 65

*Unless family history or high risk dictate otherwise.

**After 3 or more years of normal results, the Pap test may be performed less frequently at the discretion of the physician.

Source: The American College of Obstetricians and Gynecologists. Washington, D.C., and the American Cancer Society.

39. Tests maybe not to take.

Recently there have been a number of new tests that are being used for cancer screening and detection. They relate to what we call genetic testing, and are important for many women with specific risk factors for different cancers.

Some of my patients hear about these tests and they say they want them, not really understanding perhaps exactly what they are. Due to the media confusion, there is a lot of conflicting information about what these tests are for and what they can do.

For breast cancer, there is a gene called BRCA1 which was identified in 1994. Mutations in this gene are thought to account for 50% of the cases of hereditary breast cancer and 80% of hereditary ovarian cancers.* Mutations of a second gene, the BRCA2, also contribute to hereditary breast and ovarian cancers. **

It is estimated that 1 in 300 to 1 in 800 women in the United States can be genetically predisposed to BRCA1 mutations.*** Routine screening for these genes in the general population is not recommended. If a woman has a family history consistent with hereditary breast and ovarian cancer, chances of carrying a cancer predisposition gene may be as great as 50%.**

*Easton DF, Bishop DT, Ford D, et al. Genetic linkage analysis in familial breast and ovarian cancer. *Am J Hum Genet.* 1993; 52:718-722.
**Ob/Gyn Special Edition, 1999, Vol 2, A Compendium of Educational Reviews, McMahon Publishing Group, NY, NY, pages 34-35.
***Easton DF, Bishop DT, Ford D, et al. Genetic linkage analysis in familial breast and ovarian cancers: Results from 24 families. *Am J Hum Genet* 1993; 52: 671-678.

Therefore, women who have a history that raises concern over a potential hereditary cancer syndrome may be candidates for the appropriate genetic testing.*

Women with the BRCA1 mutation may have an 80%-90% lifetime risk of breast cancer, a 40%-50% lifetime risk of ovarian cancer, and a fourfold increased risk of colorectal cancer.*

Women with the BRCA2 mutation have the same lifetime risk of breast cancer, but less than a 25% lifetime risk of ovarian cancer.*

The Ashkenazi Jewish population is an exception to the general population. Approximately 1 in 50 Jewish individuals will be genetically predisposed for either a BRCA1 or BRCA2 mutation.** It is also known that Jewish women with ovarian cancer, regardless of family history, have a risk of up to 60% of harboring a BRCA1 or BRCA2 mutation.***

Now there's another gene being studied and it seems like every day something new is being discovered. It is called the hereditary nonpolyposis colorectal cancer (HNPCC) associated gene. Mutations here are related to colon cancer as well as to uterine and ovarian cancer.

*Adapted with permission from Poyner E. Cancer Screening for Women. Ob/Gyn Special Edition 1999; 2:35.

**Roa BB, Boyd AA, Volcik K, et al. Ashkenazi Jewish population frequencies for common mutations in BRCA1 and BRCA2. *Nat Genet.* 1996; 14:185-187.

***Beller U, Halle D, Cantane R, et al. High frequency of BRCA1 and BRCA2 germline mutations in Ashkenazi Jewish ovarian cancer patients, regardless of family history. *Gynecol Oncol.*. 1997; 67:123-126.

For ovarian cancer, as I said, there are no good tests, except as they relate to genetic testing I just described.

Many women request a serum CA125 or a pelvic sonogram for ovarian cancer. Unfortunately, the serum CA125 value does not achieve a high enough sensitivity or specificity to be used as a screening tool. Approximately 50% of early stage ovarian cancers will not have an elevated serum level.*

The pelvic sonogram screening does not achieve an acceptable positive predictive value for an ovarian malignancy. With this method, you would have to perform 96 surgeries before finding 4 ovarian cancers.**

So you see, not all of these tests are good for everyone.

Please consult with a physician knowledgeable about genetic testing.

*Jacobs I, Bast RC. The CA 125 tumor associated antigen: A review of the literature, *Hum Reprod.* 1989;4(1):1-12.

**Ob/Gyn Special Edition, 1999, Vol 2, A Compendium of Educational Reviews, McMahon Publishing Group, NY, NY, page 34.

40. Living well. It's not easy.

The National Institutes of Health Guidelines for exercise is 30 minutes a day, 6 days a week.

It may sound hard, but really that's light to moderate exercise. If you think about it, why do we take time to sit in front of the TV 3 hours out of the day? I mean, count, how many hours a day do people spend watching TV, every day of the week?

So why can't they sit there and do some exercise? That's right. The treadmill or the bicycle, stretching, yoga. Why do we make time to watch that favorite show for 2 hours on Thursday night and not take 30 minutes to take care of ourselves?

Some women say, "Well, I work all day without a lunch break. When I get home I'm too tired.. Just give me a diet pill!"

Life should be so easy as to take a pill.

If you put aside that 30 minutes a day as your own time, that's good medicine.

That's what I try to tell women. Everyone says they're too busy, but I try to help them to be unbusy! Organize your time!

You're going to feel busier and more hectic in your life if you don't take this time to take care of yourself.

I think exercise is very, very important, not just for your body, but for your mental outlook.

A lot of women look at eating as a way of relieving stress, but it causes stress in the long run if you put on a lot of weight!

Exercising gives you a little sense of control over yourself.

Regular weight bearing exercise is good, like walking and even dancing.

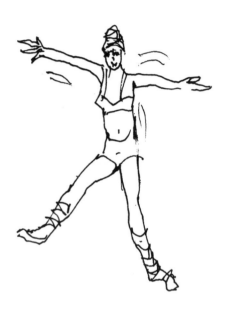

Everybody has 30 minutes a day, maybe walk to work instead of drive, or take the stairs instead of the elevator. And you know what? It's work to stay healthy!

You have to start getting into good habits, make them a normal part of your life and be proud of them.

41. Don't smoke.

You could start with this reason for not smoking:

Coronary heart disease is the biggest killer of women in the United States, and cigarette smoking doubles the risk.

Or these reasons: The carbon monoxide in cigarettes slows the transfer of oxygen from the blood to the body. The nicotine in cigarettes increases the heart rate by 15-25 beats per minute and blood pressure goes up by 15-25 points.*

Smoking also increases the risk for hypertension and brain hemorrhage.

Women who are heavy smokers are 24 times more likely to develop lung cancer than those who have never smoked. Lung cancer is the leading cause of cancer death among women, exceeding even breast cancer.*

I've spoken to teenagers about smoking, how they shouldn't start, but some of them are smoking already. They keep smoking because they don't realize they are addicted.

It's really hard for teenagers to see these things. They're so young, and they can't think of anything like getting sick or dying, not for themselves. Now it seems they could run an extra risk of damage from starting to smoke at so young an age.

*American Medical Women's Association, on line, updated March 31, 1999, page 2.

After 1 or 2 years of not smoking, your risk of heart attack drops sharply. Gradually, after about 10 years, the risk factor returns to normal.*

The risk of cancer is gradually reduced too, coming close to that of nonsmokers after 10-15 years.*

I tease the teenagers, and say it takes so long to smoke a cigarette, maybe 10 minutes, so that's 200 minutes you've wasted smoking a pack of them.

I don't want to fool with my patients. They're adults, they all have people who depend on them, and they should know better.

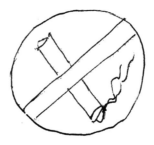

*American Medical Women's Association, on line, updated March 31, 1999, page 4.

42. Look out for fat!

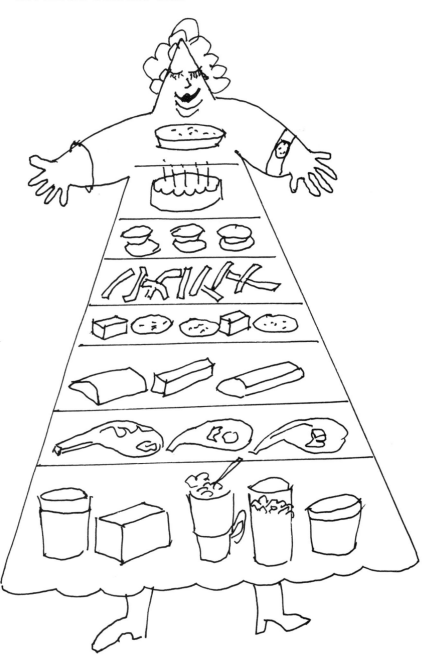

There's actually enough scientific evidence to suggest that about one-third of the cancer deaths that occur in the United States each year are due to a bad diet. Another third is due to cigarette smoking. Beyond that, many of the 1 million skin cancers that are expected to be diagnosed could have been prevented by protection from the sun's rays.*

So just think! How healthy those Americans are who don't use tobacco, who eat well, and wear sun screen.

Although genetics may be a factor in the development of cancer, behavioral factors like these, and also exercise, modify the risk of cancer at all stages of its development.

Let's go back to the turn of the century, when women were barely living beyond menopause. What were they dying of then?

Heart disease has been fairly constant, in the high range of 25% or so. But cancer hardly made the mortality charts in 1900!

The biggest killers then were pneumonia, influenza, tuberculosis, diphtheria and typhoid!*

Now we've controlled these infectious diseases. But look at that cancer.

Look what we're doing!

*Historical Statistics of the United States Colonial Times to 1970, Part 1, U.S. Department of Commerce Bureau of the Census, September 1975, page 58.

Was their diet as poor as ours? Stews and baked potatoes sound better than all that refined food and fried food we eat.

Now I must explain to women I see that a healthful diet would include 2 pieces of fruit a day, (but fruit juice doesn't count), and 3 servings of vegetables. Perhaps a daily portion of fish or chicken, and very little red meat. Nix on the fats and plenty of grains!

Think of the choices of food we have. We're too lucky! How can you say, "No!" to chocolate cake?

We really should have started good eating habits in our teens, or earlier. When you get closer to menopause, or perimenopause, your body is less forgiving of bad eating habits. The extra weight is even harder to lose.

So look out for fat!

Packaged food labels now carry nutritional facts which are very clear to read.

You should know that based on a 2,000 calorie diet, 65 grams of fat is all that is recommended for daily consumption.*

What that means is just one delicious serving of pie a la mode, and that's it for the day!

*ACOG Patient Education Brochure #AP101, July, 1995.

43. The medicine cabinet.

A patient spoke to me about all the medicine she's been taking to stay healthy. There's this image in my head of a medicine cabinet filled with calcium supplements, multivitamins, maybe something for cholesterol, or osteoporosis, then a vaginal moisturizing cream, hormones...And she doesn't even have a disease!

And her medicine cabinet begins to look funny, it's getting fuller. It's not just toothpaste and make-up anymore.

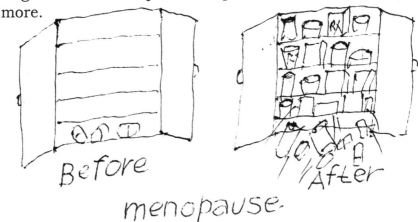

Before / After
menopause.

She never took a pill up until now, and I think a lot of women, if they never took a pill before, wonder, "Why do I have to start now?"

We may laugh at the things women take after menopause, but we have tremendous support and we should use it. The choices we have, many women in other parts of the world can't even imagine. Many don't live to be old enough to experience menopause.

We have many options to help women through this time of perimenopause, menopause and beyond. They should take advantage of that.

Be well, ask questions, and take what you need to stay well! Speak about your options with your physician who has fully examined you and is aware of your own personal history.

Preventive medicine is the key to a woman's productive longevity. That's what life is all about. Living long, but staying healthy. And being happy.

I wish everyone would understand how fortunate we are. Take advantage of it, instead of wallowing in some bad feeling, saying, "I'm having these mood swings and I want to kill someone," or, "I may be getting older and things are not going as planned." Instead, say, "I can do something" and learn how to manage your problems better and do what's good for you.

Be responsible! Fill up the medicine cabinet if you have to, even if maybe you don't want to.

What I have been telling women is that this is a time when there are a lot of changes in their bodies, and in fact women weren't meant to be alive 30 or 40 years after menopause. We all have to be careful.

When you cross the street you look both ways. Why not be just as cautious for your well-being now?